The Mediterranean Diet for Happiness

50 Enjoyable Recipes that Will Help You Eliminate Bad Eating Habits

By

Spoons of happiness

In no way is it legal to reproduce, duplicate, or transmit any part of this document in either electronic means or in printed format. Recording of this publication is strictly prohibited and any storage of this document is not allowed unless with written permission from the publisher. All rights reserved.

The information provided herein is stated to be truthful and consistent, in that any liability, in terms of inattention or otherwise, by any usage or abuse of any policies, processes, or directions contained within is the solitary and utter responsibility of the recipient reader. Under no circumstances will any legal responsibility or blame be held against the publisher for any reparation, damages, or monetary loss due to the information herein, either directly or indirectly.

Respective authors own all copyrights not held by the publisher.

The information herein is offered for informational purposes solely and is universal as so. The presentation of the information is without contract or any type of guarantee assurance.

The trademarks that are used are without any consent, and the publication of the trademark is without permission or backing by the trademark owner. All trademarks and brands within this book are for clarifying purposes only and are owned by the owners themselves, not affiliated with this document.

Table of Contents

Introduction

People always want to be happy and their searching is most of the time based on external things and situations without considering the activities they do every day.

One habit that plays an important role in people's mood is eating. The kind of food you eat can affect the way you feel. It is shown that food with high quantities of sugar and saturated fats can cause irritation and even mental disorders such as depression and anxiety.

On the contrary, plant-based food, whole grains, nuts, and fish can positively affect your mood and also your brain's functions.

This cookbook provides you 50 easy-prepared recipes to feel happy for life.

Chapter 1: Breakfast Recipes

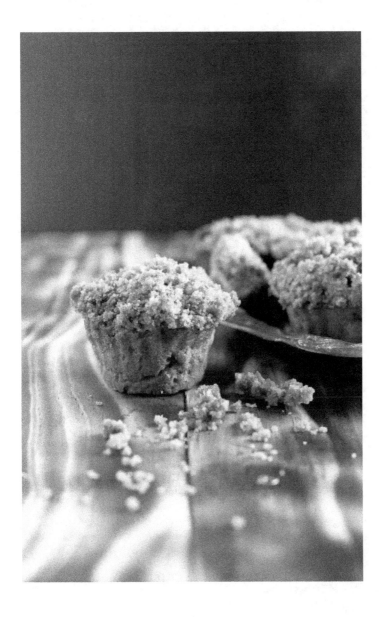

1. Muffins with Carrots

Ready in 10 minutes | Servings: 5 | Difficulty: Hard

Ingredients:

- One and 1/2 cups of whole wheat flour

- 1/2 a cup of stevia

- 1 tsp powder for baking

- 1/2 cinnamon teaspoon powder

- 1/2 tsp of soda for baking

- 1/4 cup of natural juice of apples

- Olive oil about 1/4 cup

- 1 single egg

- Fresh cranberries 1 cup

- Two carrots, grated

- Ginger 2 tsp, brushed

- 1/4 cup of chopped pecans

- Spray for cooking

Directions:

1. Combine the flour and the stevia in a big bowl, baking powder, baking soda, and Cinnamon and mix properly.

2. Include apple juice, oil, cranberries, carrots, cranberries, ginger, and pecans. But very well shake.

3. Gunk a cooking spray muffin pan, split the muffin mixture, put it in the oven, and bake it for thirty min at 375 ° Fahrenheit

4. Split among plates the muffins and serve for breakfast. Love!

Nutrition:

Calories 212, fat 3, fiber 6, carbs 14, protein 6

2. Oatmeal Pineapple

Ready in 10 minutes | Cook time: 25 minutes |
Servings: 4 | Difficulty: Normal

Ingredients:

- Old-fashioned oats with 2 cups

- 1 cup of sliced walnuts

- 2 cups of cut into cubes pineapple

- 1 tablespoon of grated ginger,

- Two cups of milk that is non-fat

- Two Eggs

- Stevia 2 teaspoons

- 2 tsp extracts of vanilla

Directions:

1. Integrate the oats with the pineapple, walnuts, and ginger in a dish. Mix and split into Four ramekins.

2. Integrate the Milk with the eggs, stevia, and vanilla in a mug, shake well and pour over the blend of oats.

3. Put it in the oven and bake it for 25 minutes at 400 ° Fahrenheit

4. For breakfast, serve. Love!

Nutrition:

Calories 211, fat 2, fiber 4, carbs 14, protein 6

3. Muffins with Spinach

Ready in 10 minutes | Servings: 6 | Difficulty: Normal

Ingredients:

- Six Eggs

- 1/2 cup milk that is non-fat

- 1 cup of low fat, collapsed cheese

- Spinach 4 ounces

- 1/2 cup red pepper roast, minced

- Prosciutto Two ounces, sliced

- Spray cooking

Directions:

1. Integrate the eggs with the milk, cheese, spinach, and red spinach in a dish. Mix well with pepper and prosciutto.

2. Oil a cooking spray muffin tray, split the muffin mix, put them in the oven, and bake for thirty min at 350 ° Fahrenheit

3. Split the plates and serve them for breakfast. Enjoy!

Nutrition:

Calories 155, fat 10, fiber 1, carbs 4, protein 10

4. Breakfast Blend for Chia Seeds

Ready in 8 hours | Servings: 4 |Difficulty: Normal

Ingredients:

- Old-fashioned oats with 2 cups

- Four tablespoons of Seeds of Chia

- Four tablespoons of sugar from coconut

- THREE cups of coconut milk

- 1 lemon zest tsp, grinded

- Blueberries 1 cup

Directions:

1. Integrate the oats with the chia seeds, sugar, milk, lemon, and chia seeds in a cup. Mix the zest and blueberries, split them into cups, and keep them in the fridge. For eight hours.

2. For breakfast, serve. Enjoy!

Nutrition:

Calories 283, fat 12, fiber 3, carbs 13, protein 8

5. Fruit Dishes for Breakfast

Ready in 10 minutes | Servings: 2 | Difficulty: Easy

Ingredients:

- One mango cup, chopped

- One sliced banana

- Pineapple, 1 cup, chopped

- One cup of milk with almonds

Directions:

1. Integrate the mango with almond milk banana, pineapple, and Stir, split into tiny bowls and offer for breakfast. Enjoy!

Nutrition:

Calories 182, fat 2, fiber 4, carbs 12, protein 6

6. Cookies for Pumpkin Breakfast

Ready in 10 minutes |Servings: 6|Difficulty: Normal

Ingredients:

- Two cups of flour of whole wheat

- Old-fashioned oats for 1 cup

- One teaspoon of soda for baking

- One pumpkin pie spice teaspoon

- Pumpkin puree for 15 ounces

- One cup of melted coconut oil

- One cup of sugar from coconut

- One single egg

- 1/2 cup of roasted pepitas, roasted

- 1/2 cup of cherries, dried-up

Directions:

1. Combine the flour with the oats, baking soda, pumpkin Spices, pumpkin puree, eggs, pepitas and cherries, oil, sugar, blend Well, out of that whole combination, form moderate cookies, place them all on a lined sheet pan in the oven and bake at 350 Degrees F. For 25 minutes

2. For breakfast, offer the cookies. Enjoy!

Nutrition:

Calories 281, fat 12, fiber 3, carbs 14, protein 6

Chapter 2: Side Dishes & Appetizer

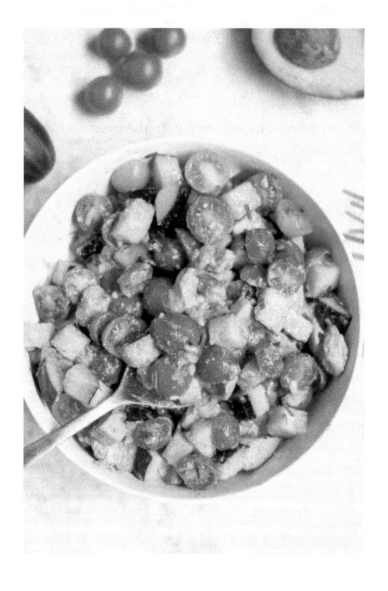

7. Avocado Salad and Tomato

Ready in 10 minutes | **Servings:** 4 | Difficulty: Normal

Ingredients:

- One minced cucumber

- Tomatoes, one pound, diced

- Two avocados, pitted, sliced, and trimmed

- One tiny red onion, cut

- Olive oil two tablespoons

- Lemon Juice 2 teaspoons

- 1/4 cup coriander, chopped

- To the taste, black pepper

Directions:

1. Comb the tomatoes with the onion, avocado, cucumber, and cilantro in a salad bowl.

2. Place the oil with the lemon juice and black pepper in a shallow saucepan, stir properly, spill over the salad, shake, and serve as a side dish.

Nutrition:

Calories 120, fat 2, fiber 2mg, carbs 3mg, protein 4g

8. Greek Salad on the Side

Ready in 10 minutes | **Servings:** 4 | Difficulty:
Normal

Ingredients:

- Sliced four pounds of heirloom tomatoes

- One yellow bell pepper, finely sliced

- One green bell pepper, finely sliced

- One red onion, finely sliced

- To the taste of black pepper

- Oregano 1/2 teaspoon, dried

- Two teaspoons of minced mint leaves

- A sprinkling of olive oil

Directions:

1. Comb the yellow and green peppers, tomatoes, onion, salt salad bowl, and pepper, toss to cover, and let stand for ten minutes.

2. Include oregano, mint, and olive oil and serve as a side salad.

Nutrition:

Calories 100, fat 2, fiber 2mg, carbs 3mg, protein 6g

9. Salad with Cucumber

Ready in 10 minutes | **Servings:** 4 | Difficulty: Normal

Ingredients:

- Two Diced English cucumbers

- Pitted and cut 8 dates

- 3/4 of a cup of fennel, cut

- Chives 2 teaspoons, chopped

- 1/2 cup of sliced walnuts

- Lemon Juice 2 teaspoons

- Four teaspoons of olive oil

- To the taste of black pepper

Directions:

1. Mix the dates, chives, fennel, lemon juice, walnuts, oil, and black pepper in a salad bowl, mix, split across plates, and serve as a side dish.

Nutrition:

Calories 100, fat 1, fiber 1mg, carbs 7mg, protein 6g

10. Side Salad with Black Beans and Vegetables

Ready in 10 minutes | **Servings:** 4 | Difficulty: Easy

Ingredients:

- One broad cucumber, sliced into chunks

- 15 ounces of dried, no-salt-added, drained, and rinsed black beans

- One cup of maize

- One cup of tomatoes with cherry, halved

- One small red, chopped onion

- Olive oil 3 tablespoons

- Four and 1/2 teaspoons of marmalade with orange

- To the taste, black pepper

- 1/2 cumin teaspoon, ground

- 1 tablespoon of Juice from a lemon

Directions:

1. Comb the beans with corn, cucumber, onion, and tomatoes in a dish.

2. Place the marmalade with oil, black pepper, lemon juice to taste, and cumin in another cup, brush, pour over the salad, toss & offer as a side dish.

Nutrition:

Calories 110, fat 0, fiber 3mg, carbs 6mg, protein 8g

11. Endives and Side Salad Escarole

Ready in 10 minutes | **Servings:** 4 | Difficulty: Normal

Ingredients:

- One shallot teaspoon, minced

- 1⁄4 cup of cider vinegar for apples

- 1 tsp Mustard from Dijon

- Three Belgian endives, minced randomly

- 3⁄4 cup of olive oil

- 1 cup of broken escarole leaves

Directions:

1. Comb escarole leaves with endives, vinegar, shallot, mustard, and oil in a pan, turn, distribute between dishes and serve as a side salad.

Nutrition:

Calories 100, fat 1, fiber 3mg, carbs 6mg, protein 7g

12. Lettuce Side Salad and Radicchio

Ready in 10 minutes | **Servings:** 4 | Difficulty: Easy

Ingredients:

- Olive oil, 1/2 cup

- To the taste, black pepper

- Shallot, 2 teaspoons, minced

- Mustard 1/4 cup

- Juice containing 2 lemons

- 1/2 cup of basil, diced

- 5 heads of baby romaine lettuce, chopped

- Three Radicchios, sliced

- Three endives, sliced roughly

Directions:

1. Comb the romaine lettuce with the radicchio and endives in a salad bowl.

2. Place the pepper, mustard, shallot, lemon juice, and basil oil in another cup, shake, add to the salad, swirl and serve as a side salad.

Nutrition:

Calories 120, fat 2, fiber 1mg, carbs 8mg, protein 2g

Chapter 3: Vegetarian and

Vegan Recipes

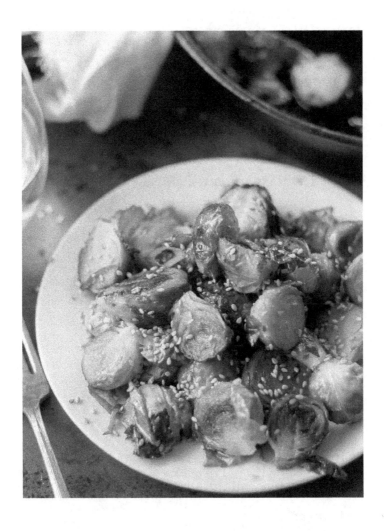

13. Sweet & Sour Brussel Sprouts

Ready in 10 minutes | Servings 2 | Difficulty: Normal

Ingredients:

- One cup sprouts from Brussel, cut

- One teaspoon of honey solvent

- 1 white pepper teaspoon

- Low-sodium, 3 tbsp soy sauce

- One tablespoon of olive oil, one tablespoon of pumpkin seeds, minced

Directions:

1. Warm the pan with olive oil.

2. Include the sliced sprouts from Brussels and roast for ten minutes. Frequently, mix the vegetables.

3. Spray them with white pepper, soy sauce, and liquid honey after that. Mix well and cook the vegetables for three minutes.

4. Connect the pumpkin seeds and blend well with them.

5. Cook the meal for an extra two minutes.

Nutrition:

109 calories, 5.3g protein, 7.7g carbohydrates, 7.3g fat, 1.9g fiber

14. Baked Tempeh

Ready in 10 minutes |Servings 6|Difficulty: Normal

Ingredients:

- Tempeh 1-pound, cubed

- 1/4 cup of low-sodium tamarium chloride

- One tsp dietary yeast

Directions:

1. Combine the tamari with nutritional yeast.

2. And roll the cubes of tempeh in the fluid and move them to a baking tray lined with a baking sheet.

3. Bake at 385F for fifteen minutes. After five minutes of cooking, turn the pieces of tempeh on the other side.

Nutrition:

154 calories, 14.8g protein, 8.3g carbohydrates, 8.2g fat, 0.2g fiber

15. Marinated Tofu

Ready in 20 minutes | Servings 3 | Difficulty: Normal

Ingredients:

- Firm tofu 10 oz, cut into cubes

- Olive oil 1 tbsp

- 1 tbsp vinegar rice

- 1 tsp of Italian seasonings

- 1 tablespoon sauce with marinara

- 1 tsp coconut oil

- 1/2 teaspoon flakes of chili

Directions:

1. Comb the rice vinegar, olive oil, the Italian seasonings, and the marinara sauce together to

produce the marinade. Apply the chili flakes and brush lightly into the mixture.

2. Then mix the marinade with the tofu pieces and keep in the fridge for 10-15 minutes.

3. In the meantime, warm the pan with coconut oil.

4. Place the marinated tofu in one layer in the pan and roast on each side for two minutes or until the cubes of tofu are light brown.

Nutrition:

132 calories, 7.8g protein, 2.5g carbohydrates, 10.7g fat, 1g fiber

16. Zucchanoush

Ready in 10 minutes | Servings 6 | Difficulty: Normal

Ingredients:

- Four zucchinis, sliced

- Olive oil Two tablespoons

- One tsp Harissa

- 1 tbsp of paste for tahini

- 1 tbsp of roasted pine nuts,

- 1/4 teaspoon crushed garlic

- 1/2 teaspoon of mint that is dried

Directions:

1. To 365 F, preheat the oven.

2. In the cookie sheet, put the zucchini, spray with olive oil and bake in the oven for thirty minutes or until the vegetables are tender.

3. Therefore, the zucchini is moved to the mixing bowl.

4. Include garlic powder, harissa, pine, nuts tahini paste, and dry mint.

5. Mix the dish, so it's smooth.

Nutrition:

123 calories, 3.2g protein, 8.1g carbohydrates, 10.1g fat, 2.6g fiber

17. Garden Stuffed Squash

Ready in 15 minutes | Servings 2 | Difficulty: Normal

Ingredients:

- 12 oz squash with butternut, cut in half

- 1 pepper bell, minced

- Leek 5 oz, diced

- One dry sage tsp

- One tablespoon coconut oil

- Two lb. mozzarella mushroom, sliced

Directions:

1. In the pot, heat the coconut oil.

2. Include the leek and bell pepper. For three minutes, roast the vegetables.

3. Insert dry sage after this and combine well.

4. Cover the vegetable combination with the butternut squash and cover with vegan Mozzarella.

5. For thirty minutes, bake the squash halves at 360 F.

Nutrition:

289 calories, 4.4g protein, 41.6g carbohydrates, 13.4g fat, 5.6g fiber

Chapter 4: Poultry Recipes

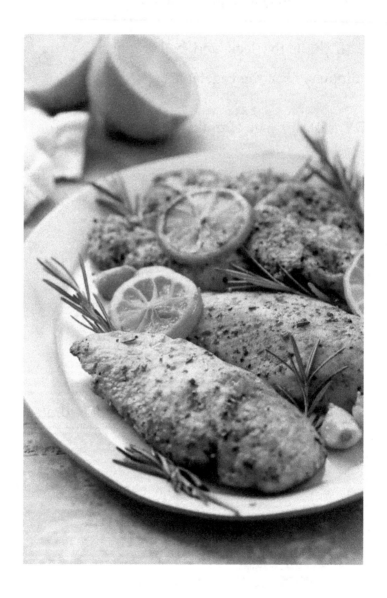

18. Rosemary Roasted Chicken

Ready in 1 hour and 20 minutes | Servings 8 | Difficulty: Normal

Ingredients:

- One chicken

- One clove of garlic, diced

- One tbsp chopped rosemary

- Olive oil 1 tablespoon

- For the taste, black pepper

- Eight springs of rosemary

Directions:

1. Place the garlic with the rosemary in a cup, scrub the chicken with the black pepper, combine the oil with the rosemary, put it in a baking dish, place it in the oven at 350 ° F with the roast for 1 hour and 20 minutes.

2. Carve chicken, split between plates, and serve with a side salad.

Nutrition:

Calories 325, fat 5g, fiber 1mg, carbs 15mg, protein 14g

19. Chicken, Scallions and Carrot Mix

Ready in 10 minutes | Servings 6 | Difficulty: Easy

Ingredients:

- Four cups of fried, skinless, boneless, and ripped chicken

- Olive oil 1/4 cup

- Balsamic vinegar 1/3 cup

- One tiny red head of cabbage, ripped

- 1 cup of grated carrot

- Six scallions, in slices

- To the taste, black pepper

Directions:

1. Combine the olive oil and vinegar in a cup and shake.

2. Comb the chicken with the black pepper scallions, cabbage, and carrot in a salad dish.

3. Include the combination of vinegar and oil, swirl, and serve.

Nutrition:

Calories 170, fat 2g, fiber 2mg, carbs 12mg, protein 6g

20. Chicken Sandwich

Ready in 16 minutes | Servings 4 | Difficulty: Easy

Ingredients:

- Four breasts of chicken

- 1/2 Italian seasoning teaspoon

- One eggplant, cut finely

- To the taste, black pepper

- A sprinkling of olive oil

- 1/2 cup tomato sauce with reduced sodium

- Sixteen leaves of basil, ripped

- Eight ounces of low-fat cheese with mozzarella, shredded

- Eight bread slices of whole wheat

Directions:

1. Add a sprinkling of oil to the chicken, brush with black pepper to taste, and scatter with the Italian seasoning.

2. Over medium-high fire, burn up a grill, introduce chicken, cook on either side for five minutes, switch off the heat, and set aside for now.

3. Season the black pepper eggplant slices to taste, position them on a hot grill, and bake on each side for three minutes.

4. Arrange 2 slices of bread on a work board, put 1 ounce of mozzarella cheese on each slice of bread, put two slices of eggplant on one slice, One piece of grilled chicken, two tablespoons of tomato sauce, Four leaves of basil, and cover with the other slice of bread.

5. For the rest of the bread slices and the remainder of the ingredients, replicate this, split them between plates, and serve.

Nutrition:

Calories 200, fat 2g, fiber 6mg, carbs 14mg, protein 12 mg

21. Chicken Tortillas

Ready in 10 | Servings 4 | Difficulty: Easy

Ingredients:

- Four tortillas of whole wheat, cooked up

- 1/3 cup yogurt free from fat

- Six ounces of skinless, boneless chicken breasts, baked and sliced into

- Strips

- Two tomatoes, diced

- To the taste, black pepper

Directions:

1. Heat a skillet over medium heat, introduce one tortilla at a time, heat it up, and put it up on a working surface.

2. On each tortilla, layer yogurt, add chicken & tomatoes, roll, split between plates, and serve.

Nutrition:

Calories 190, fat 2g, fiber 2mg, carbs 12mg, protein 6g

22. Chicken Cream

Ready in 20 minutes | Servings 4 | Difficulty: Normal

Ingredients:

- Two breasts of chicken, boneless, skinless & sliced into pieces

- One chopped yellow onion

- Olive oil, 2 tablespoons

- One clove of garlic, diced

- Twelve ounces of zucchini, in cubes

- Two bits of carrots, minced

- To the taste, black pepper

- Fourteen ounces of coco-milk

- Seventeen ounces of chicken stock with reduced sodium

Directions:

1. Over medium-high pressure, heat a pan with the oil, add the garlic and onion, mix and simmer for five minutes.

2. Include the carrots, chicken, zucchini, chicken stock & black pepper, whisk, bring to a boil, lower the heat to mild and boil for fifteen minutes.

3. Include the milk, move the soup to the mixer, pulse, ladle into the bowls of soup and eat.

Nutrition:

Calories 210, fat 7g, fiber 4mg, carbs 15mg, protein 12mg

Chapter 5: Beef, Pork, Lamb

Recipes

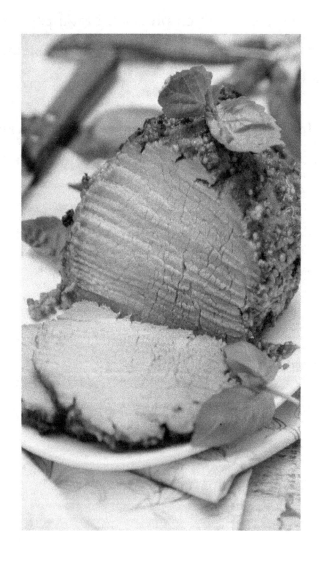

23. Spiced Beef

Ready in 80 minutes | Servings 4 | Difficulty: Easy

Ingredients:

- 1-pound sirloin of beef

- One tablespoon seasoning five-spice

- One leaf of bay

- Two Cups of Water

- One peppercorn teaspoon

Directions:

1. Brush the meat with seasoning with five spices and position it in the casserole.

2. Add nay leaves, water, and peppercorns.

3. Cover the cap and boil over medium heat for 80 minutes.

4. Chop the cooked meat and pour hot spiced water over it. From a casserole.

Nutrition:

213 calories, 34.5g protein, 0.5g carbohydrates, 7.1g fat, 0.2g fiber

24. Tomato Beef

Ready in 17 minutes |Servings 2|Difficulty: Normal

Ingredients:

- Two chuck steaks shoulder

- 1/4 cup of sauce with tomatoes

- Olive oil, 1 tablespoon

Directions:

1. Rub the tomato sauce and olive oil with the steaks and pass the grill is preheated to 390F.

2. For nine minutes, grill the beef.

3. And turn it on the other side and cook it for another 10 min.

Nutrition:

247 calories, 21.4g protein, 1.7g carbohydrates, 17.1g fat, 0.5g fiber

25. Sage Beef Loin

Ready in 18 minutes | Servings 2 | Difficulty: Normal

Ingredients:

- Ten oz loin of beef, strips

- 1 clove of garlic, diced

- Margarine two tablespoons

- One dried sage teaspoon

Directions:

1. In the pan, swirl the margarine.

2. Add the garlic and dried sage and roast on a low heat for two minutes.

3. Insert the beef loin strips as well as roast them over moderate flame for fifteen minutes. Now and then, whisk the meat.

Nutrition:

363 calories, 38.2g protein, 0.8g carbohydrates, 23.2g fat, 0.2g fiber

26. Beef Chili

Ready in 30 minutes | Servings 2 | Difficulty: Easy

Ingredients:

- One cup of lean, ground lean beef

- One slice of onion, minced

- Olive oil, 1 tablespoon

- 1 cup of tomatoes crushed

- 1/2 cup of cooked red kidney beans

- 1/2 of a cup of water

- Seasonings of 1 teaspoon chili

Directions:

1. In a frying pan, boil up the olive oil and add some lean ground beef.

2. Over medium heat, simmer for 7 minutes.

3. Then add the diced onion and chili seasonings. Combine the items and have them baked for ten minutes.

4. Add water, smashed tomatoes, red kidney beans, and whisk after this. with the chili.

5. For 13 minutes, shut the lid and boil the meal.

Nutrition:

220 calories, 18.3g protein, 22g carbohydrates, 6.7g fat, 6.1g fiber

27. Celery Beef Stew

Ready in 55 minutes | Servings 3 | Difficulty: Hard

Ingredients:

- 1-pound loin of beef, sliced

- Celery stalk, two cups, diced

- One clove of garlic, diced

- 1 onion in purple, diced

- Olive oil, 1 tbsp

- 1 tbsp of paste with tomato

- 1 chili powder teaspoon

- 1 dry dill teaspoon

- Two Cups of Water

Directions:

1. Fry the beef loin in a saucepan for five minutes with olive oil.

2. Insert all the rest of the ingredients afterward, and close the lid.

3. On medium fire, cook the stew for 50 minutes.

Nutrition:

150 calories, 14.6g protein, 4.6g carbohydrates, 7.9g fat, 1.2g fiber

Chapter 6: DASH Diet

Seafood Recipes

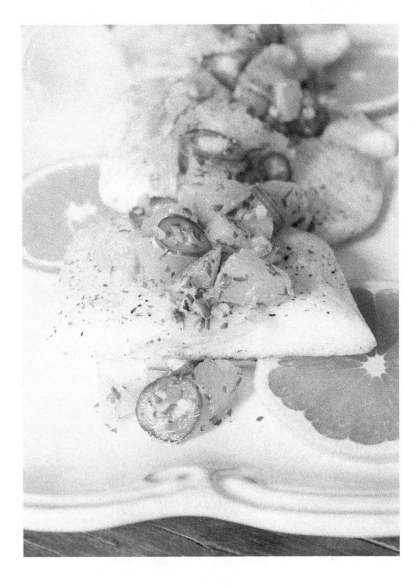

28. Halibut with Radish Slices

Ready in 10 min| Servings: 2| Difficulty: Normal.

Ingredients:

- 4 halibut fillets, boneless

- 1 cup radishes, sliced

- 1 tablespoon apple cider vinegar

- ¼ teaspoon ground coriander

- 1 tablespoon olive oil

- 1 teaspoon low-fat cream cheese

Directions:

1. Sprinkle apple cider vinegar, ground coriander, and olive oil with the fish fillets.

2. Then grill the halibut for 3 minutes per side in the preheated to 385F fire.

3. Move the fish to the plates and finish with the cream cheese and sliced radish.

Nutrition:

356 calories,60.8g protein, 1g carbohydrates, 10.5g fat, 0.5g fiber, 94mg cholesterol, 170mg sodium, 1378mg potassium

29. Green Onion Salmon

Ready in 10 minutes | Servings: 4 | Difficulty: Normal.

Ingredients:

- 4 green olives, pitted, sliced

- 2 oz. green onions, blended

- ½ teaspoon chili flakes

- ¼ teaspoon ground black pepper

- 3 tablespoons avocado oil

- 4 salmon fillets, skinless and boneless

- 1 oz. parsley, chopped

Directions:

1. Mix the green onions, chili flakes, ground black pepper, avocado oil, and parsley.

2. Then rub the green onion mixture with the salmon fillets and pass them into the preheated skillet.

3. Cook it on one side for 4 minutes.

4. Cover with sliced olives on the fried cod.

Nutrition:

Per serving: 272 calories, 35.1g protein, 3.2g carbohydrates, 13.4g fat, 1.1g fiber, 78mg cholesterol, 375mg sodium, 797mg potassium

30. Broccoli and Cod Mash

Ready in 10 min| Servings: 2| Difficulty: Normal.

Ingredients:

- 2 cups broccoli, chopped

- 4 cod fillets, boneless, chopped

- 1 white onion, chopped

- 2 tablespoons olive oil

- 1 cup of water

- 1 tablespoon low-fat cream cheese

- ½ teaspoon ground black pepper

Directions:

1. In a saucepan, roast the cod with olive oil for 1 minute on either side.

2. Then, except for the cream cheese, add all the other ingredients and cook the meal for 18 minutes.

3. Drain the bath, add the cream cheese, and cook the meal well after that.

Nutrition:

186 calories,21.8g protein, 5.8g carbohydrates, 9.1g fat, 1.8g fiber, 43mg cholesterol, 105mg sodium, 191mg potassium

31. Greek Style Salmon

Ready in 10 min| Servings: 2| Difficulty: Normal.

Ingredients:

- 4 medium salmon fillets, skinless and boneless

- 1 tablespoon lemon juice

- 1 tablespoon dried oregano

- 1 teaspoon dried thyme

- ¼ teaspoon onion powder

- 1 tablespoon olive oil

Directions:

1. Heat olive oil in the skillet.

2. Sprinkle the salmon with dried oregano, thyme, onion powder, and lemon juice.

3. Put the fish in the skillet and cook for 4 minutes per side.

Nutrition:

271 calories, 34.7g protein, 1.1g carbohydrates, 14.7g fat, 0.6g fiber, 78mg cholesterol, 80mg sodium, 711mg potassium

32. Spicy Ginger Seabass

Ready in 10 min| Servings: 2| Difficulty: Normal.

Ingredients:

- 1 tablespoon ginger, grated

- 2 tablespoons sesame oil

- ¼ teaspoon chili powder

- 4 sea bass fillets, boneless

- 1 tablespoon margarine

Directions:

1. Heat sesame oil and margarine in the skillet.

2. Add chili powder and ginger.

3. Then add seabass and cook the fish for 3 minutes per side.

4. Then close the lid and simmer the fish for 3 minutes over low heat.

Nutrition:

216 calories,24g protein, 1.1g carbohydrates, 12.3g fat, 0.2g fiber, 54mg cholesterol, 123mg sodium, 354mg potassium

Chapter 7: DASH Diet Soup

and Stew Recipes

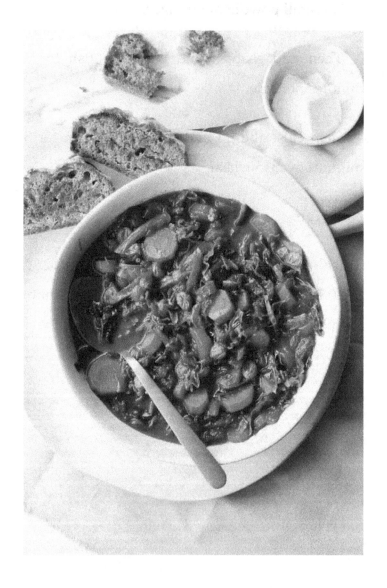

33. Red Cabbage Soup

Ready in 40 minutes | Servings 4 | Difficulty Normal

Ingredients:

- Red cabbage 1-pound, shredded

- One chopped yellow onion

- Olive oil, 1 tablespoon

- 1 tsp dry oregano

- Leek 3 oz, chopped

- Three cups of low-sodium broth for chicken

Directions:

1. Over medium heat, warm a pot with the oil, insert the onion and leek, stir and simmer for five minutes.

2. Stir in the cabbage and all the rest of the ingredients from the list above and simmer for 35 minutes over moderate flame.

Nutrition:

95 calories, 3.6g protein, 13.2g carbohydrates, 3.7g fat, 4g fiber

34. Celery and Leek Soup

Ready in 60 minutes | Servings 4 | Difficulty Hard

Ingredients:

- Celery stalk, 2 cups, diced

- One chopped yellow onion

- Olive oil, 1 tablespoon

- Flakes with 1 teaspoon with chili

- Chopped 1 cup of leek

- Three cups of low-sodium broth of chicken

- 1/2 teaspoon of sage dry

Directions:

1. Over medium-high heat, warm a pot with the oil, insert the onion, celery, and leek, mix and simmer for five minutes.

2. Include the rest of the ingredients and boil for 55 minutes to make the soup.

3. Mix the cooked soup until creamy with the electric mixer.

Nutrition:

74 calories, 2.5g protein, 8.1g carbohydrates, 3.7g fat, 1.8g fiber

35. Collard Greens Soup

Ready in 30 minutes | Servings 4 | Difficulty Normal

Ingredients:

- Four cups chicken broth low in sodium

- Chicken breast, eight ounces, boneless, skinless, and sliced

- Collard greens, two cups, sliced

- 1/2 tsp of oregano that is dried

- 1/2 of a tsp of white pepper

- 1/2 teaspoon paprika

Directions:

1. Put the chicken, oregano, white pepper, paprika, and chicken broth in a bowl. For 20 minutes, boil the products over a moderate flame.

2. Include the collard greens, then simmer for another ten minutes.

Nutrition:

88 calories, 14.6g protein, 2.7g carbohydrates, 1.6g fat, 1g fiber

36. Stalk Soup

Ready in 40 minutes | Servings 4 | Difficulty
Normal

Ingredients:

- Cauliflower florets, Two pounds

- Olive oil, 1 tablespoon

- One cup puree tomato

- One cup of diced celery

- Six cups of low-sodium broth for chicken

- New cilantro Three teaspoons, minced

- 1 tsp of powdered curry

Directions:

1. Over medium-high heat, warm a pot with the oil, introduce the celery, mix, and sauté for five minutes.

2. Apply all the rest of the ingredients after this, and boil the soup for 35 minutes.

Nutrition:

139 calories, 8.8g protein, 20.2g carbohydrates, 4g fat, 7.5g fiber

Chapter 8: Salads & Sauces

Recipes

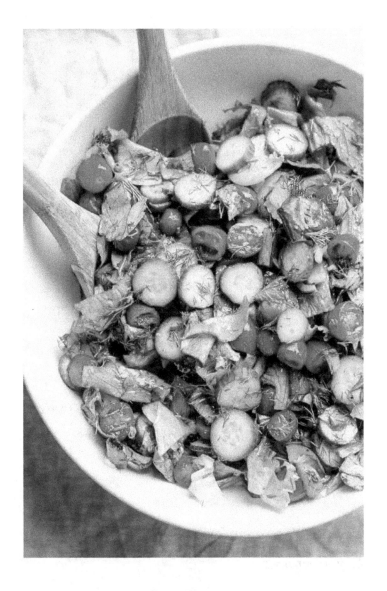

37. Cucumber and Lettuce Salad

Ready in: 5 minutes | Servings: 4 | Difficulty Easy

Ingredients:

- 1 tablespoon canola oil

- 1 cup cucumber, chopped

- ½ pound green beans, cooked, roughly chopped

- 1 cup corn kernels, cooked

- 2 cups romaine lettuce, roughly chopped

Directions:

1. Merge all the salad ingredients and cool for about 3 minutes in the refrigerator.

Nutrition:

Calories 89, protein 2.6g, carbohydrates 13.1g, fat 4.1g, fiber 3.3g.

38. Endive-Kale Salad

Ready in: 4 minutes | Servings: 4 | Difficulty
Easy

Ingredients:

- 2 cups kale, chopped

- 1 tablespoon balsamic vinegar

- 1 teaspoon sesame seeds

- 1 tablespoon sesame oil

- 2 tablespoons lime juice

- 1 head endives, chopped

Directions:

1. Place all of the ingredients listed above in the salad bowl and mix the salad well.

Nutrition:

Calories 75, protein 2.8g, carbohydrates 8.5g, fat 4.1g, fiber 4.6g.

39. Salad Skewers

Ready in: 10 minutes | Servings: 4 | Difficulty Easy

Ingredients:

- 1 teaspoon olive oil

- ½ teaspoon lemon juice

- 2 cups cherry tomatoes

- 2 cucumbers

Directions:

1. Slice the cucumbers into medium-sized cubes.

2. Then loop the cucumber and cherry tomatoes into the skewers one at a time.

3. Then spray lemon juice and olive oil on the salad skewers.

Nutrition:

Calories 49, protein 1.8g, carbohydrates 9g, fat 1.5g, fiber 1.8g.

40. Nectarine Salad with Shrimps

Ready in: 7 minutes | Servings: 4 | Difficulty Normal

Ingredients:

- ¼ teaspoon ground black pepper

- 1 teaspoon lemon juice

- 1 teaspoon margarine

- 1 tablespoon olive oil

- 6 oz shrimps, peeled

- 1 nectarine, pitted, chopped

- 1 cup spring mix salad greens

Directions:

1. In the skillet, add the margarine and heat it.

2. Mix the ground black pepper and shrimp.

3. Then put the shrimp in the hot margarine and cook on each side for about 3 minutes.

4. Place the fried shrimp in a salad dish.

5. Put the salad greens, chopped nectarines, olive oil, and lemon juice into the spring mix.

6. Give the salad a shake.

Nutrition:

Calories 110, protein 10.6g, carbohydrates 4.5g, fat 5.4g, fiber 0.9g.

41. Asian Style Cobb Salad

Ready in: 10 minutes | Servings: 4 | Difficulty Easy

Ingredients:

- 1 tablespoon lemon zest, grated

- 1 tablespoon sesame seeds

- 3 tablespoons balsamic vinegar

- 1 tablespoon avocado oil

- 1 avocado, sliced

- 3 oz scallions, chopped

- 1 cup carrot, grated

- 1 cup tangerines, peeled

- 2 cup lettuce, chopped

Directions:

1. Mix the sesame seeds, balsamic vinegar, lemon zest, and avocado oil together to create the salad dressing.

2. In the dish, put all the remaining ingredients and add the salad dressing on top.

3. Before eating, shake the salad gently.

Nutrition:

Calories 195, protein 2.5g, carbohydrates 16.3g, fat 14.5g.

Chapter 9: Lunch & Dinner

Recipes

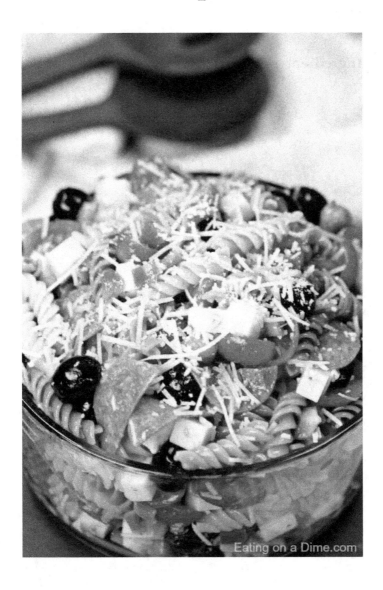

Eating on a Dime.com

42. Italian Pasta Mix

Ready in 20 minutes | Servings: 4 | Difficulty
Hard

Ingredients:

- One-pound penne pasta with whole
  wheat, cooked

- Three cloves of garlic, diced

- Olive oil, Two tablespoons

- Three carrots, cut

- One bunch of asparagus, divided into
  moderate pieces and cut

- One bell pepper red, diced

- 1 bell pepper purple, chopped

- One cup of tomatoes with raspberry,
  halved

- A squeeze of black pepper

- 2/3 cup of milk of coconut

- 2 teaspoons low-fat, grated parmesan

Directions:

1. Over medium-high heat, warm a skillet with the oil, add the garlic, stir and simmer for 2 minutes.

2. Insert the vegetables, stir and simmer for an additional four minutes.

3. Add the asparagus, mix, cover the pan, and simmer for a further eight minutes.

4. Include the bell peppers, yellow and red, and combine and roast for 5 minutes.

5. Insert black pepper, cherry tomatoes, milk, parmesan, and pasta, mix, split between plates, and eat.

Nutrition:

Calories 221, fat 4mg, fiber 4mg, carbs 15mg, protein 9mg

43. Glazed Ribs

Ready in 1 hour and 20 minutes | Servings: 4 | Difficulty Normal

Ingredients:

- One Pork rack ribs, split ribs

- One and a quarter cups of tomato sauce

- White vinegar for 1/4 cup

- Spicy Mustard for 3 tablespoons

- Two tablespoons of sugar from coconut

- Water for 3 tablespoons

- 1/4 teaspoon of warm sauce

- One onion powder tsp

- Spray for cooking

Directions:

1. Place the ribs in a baking bowl, cover them with tin foil and roast them for 1 hour at 400 °F in the oven.

2. Warm the tomato sauce, mustard, sugar, vinegar, water, onion powder, and hot sauce in a saucepan, mix, boil for ten minutes, then turn off.

3. Baste the ribs with half of this sauce, put them over medium-high heat on a hot oven rill, grease them with a cooking spray, cook on either side for four minutes, split among plates, and serve with the remaining sauce on the side.

Nutrition:

Calories 287, fat 5mg, fiber 8mg, carbs 16mg, protein 15mg

44. Pork Chops and Sauce

Ready in 9 hours | Servings: 6 | Difficulty Hard

Ingredients:

- Six chops of pork loin

- Olive oil, 1 tablespoon

- Crushed 2 tablespoons of tapioca,

- 1 minced yellow onion

- Low-sodium 10-ounce mushroom soup cream

- 1/2 cup of juice for apples

- Thyme 2 teaspoons, diced

- 1 and 1/2 cups of cut mushrooms

- 1/4 teaspoon crushed garlic

Directions:

1. Heat the oil in a pan over medium-high temperature, introduce the pork chops, brown on each side for four minutes and move to a slow cooker.

2. Include the crushed tapioca, onion, mushroom soup sauce, apple juice, thyme, mushrooms, and ground garlic.

Nutrition:

Calories 229, fat 4mg, fiber 9mg, carbs 16mg, protein 17mg

45. Shrimp and Pomegranate Sauce

Ready in 50 minutes | Servings: 4 | Difficulty Normal

Ingredients:

- 1-quart of juice for pomegranate

- 1/2 cup sugar for coconut

- 1/4 Cup of Lemon Juice

- 1 pound of Peeled and Deveined Shrimp

- 1/2 cumin seed, field

- 3/4 teaspoon of cilantro, field

- 1/4 teaspoon of dried cinnamon

- Olive oil, 1 and 1/2 teaspoons

- A squeeze of black pepper

- Four baby arugula cups

Directions:

1. Incorporate the pomegranate juice in a pan with the olive sugar and olive extract. Sugar, whisk, put over medium heat to a boil and cook for 45 Minutes.

2. Integrate the shrimp in a dish with the cumin, cinnamon, cilantro, black pepper, and oil, and mix well with it.

3. Heat up a medium-hot plate, add shrimp and cook for 2 minutes. Switch to a bowl on either side

4. Insert the pomegranate sauce and arugula, mix, and serve. For lunch.

Nutrition:

Calories 281, fat 5mg, fiber 8mg, carbs 17mg, protein 14mg

46. Eggplants and Tomatoes Mix

Ready in 25 minutes | Servings: 4 | Difficulty Normal

Ingredients:

- One purple, cubed eggplant

- Two cloves of garlic, diced

- Olive oil, 2 tablespoons

- One cumin paste, ground

- One sweet paprika teaspoon

- 1/2 cup of coriander, chopped

- 14 ounces of canned low-sodium tomatoes, diced

Directions:

1. Over medium-high heat, warm a pan with the oil, add the eggplant, stir and cook for 1 minute.

2. Add the garlic, mix, cook for 1 min, cover the skillet, decrease the heat to medium-low and cook for 10 minutes.

3. Insert paprika, cilantro, and cumin and simmer for 1 minute, stir and cook.

4. Include the tomatoes, cover with a lid and simmer for an additional ten minutes.

5. Divide and serve into containers.

Nutrition:

Calories 233, fat 3mg, fiber 7mg, carbs 16mg, protein 7mg

Chapter 10: Desserts &

Snacks

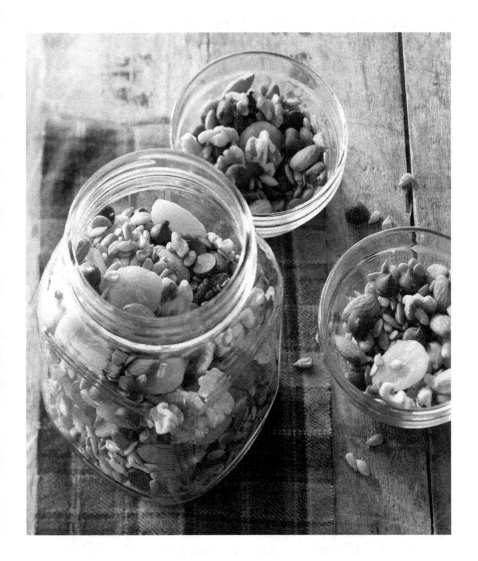

47. Nuts and Seeds Mix

Ready in 10 minutes | Servings: 6 | **Difficulty:** Easy

Ingredients:

- One Cup of a pecan

- One Cup of hazelnuts

- One mug with almonds

- 1/4 of a cup of coconut, sliced

- One Cup with walnuts

- Bits of 1/2 cup papaya, dry

- 1/2 cup, cooked, pitted, and chopped dates

- 1/2 cup of seeds of sunflower

- 1/2 cup of seeds for pumpkin

- One Cup of raisins

Directions:

1. Integrate the pecans with coconut, walnuts, papaya, hazelnuts, almonds, dates, sunflower seeds, pumpkin seeds, and raisins in a bowl, whisk them together and serve as a snack.

Nutrition:

Calories 188, fat 4mg, fiber 6mg, carbs 8mg, protein 6mg

48. Tortilla Chips

Ready in 25 minutes | Servings: 6 | **Difficulty:** Easy

Ingredients:

- 12 tortillas of whole wheat, sliced into 6 wedges each.

- Olive oil, 2 tablespoons

- 1 tablespoon of powdered chili

- A pinch of spice from Cayenne

Directions:

1. On a roasting pan, lay the tortillas, insert the oil, chili flakes, and cayenne, mix, put in the oven, and bake for 25 minutes at 350-degree Fahrenheit

2. Divide and serve as a side dish in bowls.

Nutrition:

Calories 199, fat 3mg, fiber 4mg, carbs 12mg, protein 5mg

49. Kale Chips

Ready in 15 minutes | Servings: 8 | **Difficulty:** Easy

Ingredients:

- One cluster of kale leaves

- Olive oil, One tablespoon

- 1 tsp of paprika smoked

- A squeeze of black pepper

Directions:

1. On a baking tray, scatter the kale leaves, incorporate black pepper, oil, and paprika, swirl, put in the oven, and cook at 350 degrees F for fifteen minutes.

2. Divide into bowls and serve as a snack.

Nutrition:

Calories 177, fat 2mg, fiber 4mg, carbs 13mg, protein 6mg

50. Potato Chips

Ready in 30 minutes | Servings: 6 |**Difficulty:**
Normal

Ingredients:

- Two potatoes of gold, cut into thin rounds

- Olive oil, 1 tablespoon

- Two teaspoons of garlic, diced

Directions:

1. Integrate the potato chips with the oil and garlic in a tub, mix, scatter on a rimmed baking sheet, put in the oven, and bake for thirty min at 400 ° Fahrenheit

2. Split and serve into bowls.

Nutrition:

Calories 200, fat 3g, fiber 5mg, carbs 13mg, protein 6mg

Conclusion

Many studies have found that keeping a healthy diet has plenty of benefits for everything. It can prevent chronic diseases such as cancer and cardiovascular problems, and mental health disorders like depression.

A high intake of fresh vegetables and fruits, nuts, whole grains, olive oil is related to a low risk of depression while a high intake of red meat, sugar, high-fat dairy products can lead to a risk of depression.

The Mediterranean recipes present in this cookbook are the key to maintain you healthy and happy.